The Rally Board

By Ed Sasena

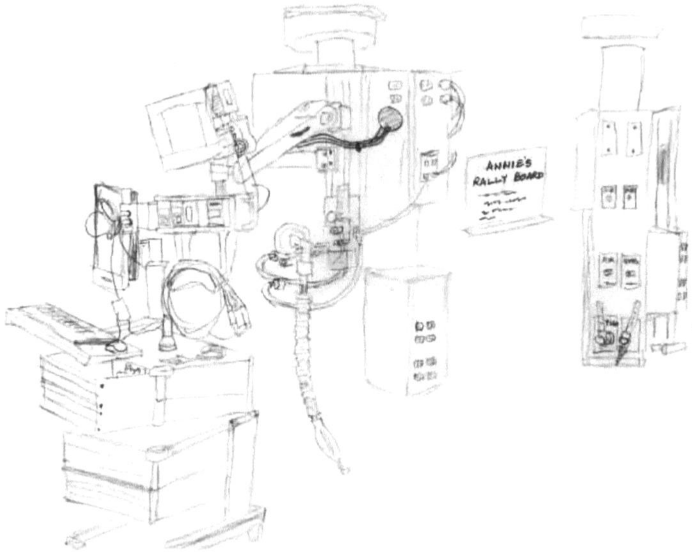

Figure 1: Sophisticated ICU Equipment Surrounding the Simple, But Powerful Rally Board

ISBN 10: 0-9785791-1-9
ISBN 13: 978-0-9785791-1-1

www.erallyboard.com

Table of Contents

Figures

Tables

Preface

The process of birth always scared me. So many things could go wrong that it seemed like a miracle that it could ever happen without anything going wrong. We experienced that miracle with the birth of our first child in 1994. With our second child, however, my fears became reality - to an extent that I never imagined.

What follows is the story of the journey our family took down the road of pediatric cardiology – a road that was simultaneously the most frightening and rewarding road any of us had traveled up to that point. The experience provided a hard lesson in properly managing our expectations in order to physically, emotionally, and mentally survive the trip.

I am documenting our experience in an attempt to provide another glimmer of hope to those that come after us. The details in this book are those that were actually generated during our experience. They are documented here to benefit those that are about to experience what we did but are not getting satisfactory answers when they ask questions about what to expect.

The hard lesson learned was that a sense of progress is an important, motivating reward in any circumstance. The more difficult the circumstance, the more difficult it becomes to find that sense of progress – especially if one does not adjust the difficulty of what one is attempting to achieve. A professional cyclist may set his or her sites on winning the Tour de France. If a beginner were to do the same, then disappointment would certainly result. But if the beginner were to attempt to achieve the absence of sore muscles prior to the next ride, then progress is almost certain. As progress is made, difficulty in the circumstance decreases allowing one to increase the difficulty of what is attempting to be accomplished.

Maintaining a strong sense of faith that the big goal can be achieved is also very important. With that faith comes the perseverance and discipline to continue keeping goals simple for as long as it takes to put together more wins than losses.

The Rally Board took on a life of its own, helping us focus on progress and communicate that progress to many, many people – first by way of a white board in our Intensive Care Unit bed space, next by way of emails sent to family and friends, then expanded email distribution to include work colleagues and people we didn't even know. Eventually, the Rally Board became a website visited by people all over the world. The Rally Board gave us a means of focusing on the simple goals and magnifying small progress beyond our wildest dreams.

What is not captured here is the overwhelming support that we received as a result of the Rally Board. That support was instrumental in our family making it through this experience intact. Hopefully, you or someone you know will have a Rally Board or some similar mechanism to help them maintain focus on the small bits of progress that are often so difficult to see when your vision is blocked by the gravity of a challenging situation.

Tedy Bruschi, NFL Football Super Bowl Champion linebacker for the New England Patriots, summed up the essence of the Rally Board as he described how he successfully recovered from a life-threatening stroke. "I tried to celebrate the small victories"[1], Bruschi said. As you will see in the pages that follow, that's what the Rally Board is all about – celebrating the small victories.

1. "You Can Get Your Life Back," Boston Sunday Globe's *Parade, The Sunday Newspaper Magazine*, September 24, 2006, pg 5.

About the Cover

The first time I stepped outside of the hospital building and walked down the street for a breath of fresh air, I was overcome with a very strange feeling. It was as if I came down from another planet to visit Earth. The streets were bustling with traffic. Sirens broke through the noise of the city. Pedestrians scurried about the sidewalks to their destinations. But no one knew about the gravity of the situation that my family and I were immersed in. Our lives were somewhat stalled yet life went on without us. How I wished I could have traded problems with any one of the people on that street – even if it were just for one day. Then an important lesson began to sink deep into me. Don't take life or the people around you for granted. "Don't sweat the small stuff," as they say. Many of the worries that the people on that street were dragging around with them could easily have been left behind.

Six years later we were walking in the American Heart Association's annual Heart Walk. This year's Walk had a very special twist to it, however. Over one hundred advertising banners had been hung all over the city along the Walk route. There, on every banner, larger than life, was a photo from last year's walk of my daughter sitting on my shoulders!

Seeing the banners brought back the vivid memories of that walk down the street near the hospital six years earlier. Here were all of these photos of my daughter and me, yet no one was paying attention to them. Life was going on all around us just like it was six years earlier. It was a good reminder of the lesson learned earlier. Although during this year's Heart Walk, a sense of inspiration came over me. Despite the fact that people weren't really paying attention to the banners, there were thousands of people walking past them who cared enough to raise money for the cause and take time out of their weekend to make a difference. We are not alone. There are many families out there like ours and even more that want to help.

Credits

Thanks to the following people for their help in getting this book off of my computer and into a format that can be helpful to others.

- "A Nurse's Perspective" provided by Suzanne Murphy McDonough, R.N./BSN.
- Logistical support provided by Heather Sheldon and Matt Berg.
- Editorial advice provided by Chris Hirshland, Matt Berg, and my wife.
- Photography provided by my wife and Elizabeth Muff.
- Illustrations provided by my daughter and me.
- Moral support provided by my wife, children, family, friends, and colleagues

Special thanks to all of the doctors, nurses, administrative staff, and volunteers at the Hospital who devote their time to bringing about monumental changes in the lives of so many families.

Dedication

This book is dedicated to the memory of a little girl who went into the Fontan surgery at the same time that Annie did. After opening her chest, the doctors decided that the surgery was too risky to complete. She and her family endured the same recovery process that we did without the benefit of completing the task at hand.

Four years later in April, 2004, she was given the option of trying again. After weighing the risks of surgery against the risk of complications endured by not having the surgery, she bravely chose to proceed. Although she made it through surgery, she didn't survive the recovery and passed away at the age of 11.

May we all have half the courage that she had. God bless A.G.

The Rally Board

MAY 1997 - DOWN, UP, DOWN SYNDROME

Although my wife was having a seemingly normal pregnancy, our OB had suggested that she have an amniocentesis performed due to slightly high readings from the alpha feto protein test. During the amniocentesis procedure an ultrasound was performed to direct the insertion of the needle. The technician noticed something peculiar. My wife sensed that they were concerned about something but nothing was mentioned due to initial uncertainties. She was in her sixteenth week of pregnancy at the time of the procedure.

A few weeks later, our regular OB visit began with a meeting in his office - a sign that my wife's suspicions were correct. He obviously did not have good news for us. They detected an abnormal measurement of the nuchal fold which is the skin on the back side of the fetus' neck. From a top view of the skull the distance between the outside of the skull and the outside of the skin should measure no more than 6 mm. Although the OB did not give a conclusive diagnosis, he said that he has never seen this condition indicate anything other than Down Syndrome. He expected that the results of the chromosome analysis would indicate the presence of Down Syndrome. We spent the next two days in miserable depression digesting the news.

Late on a Friday night we received a very encouraging but still inconclusive phone message at home from the OB. Results from 4 of the 15 cells being analyzed indicated that Down Syndrome was not present. Chances of this being the final result were very good. Hesitant to get our hopes up too much, the weight of the world seemed to fall off of our shoulders throughout the course of the weekend. Nevertheless, the OB still wanted us to report on Monday morning to the Prenatal Diagnostic Center for a check up by a specialist.

On Monday morning, the specialist, along with his assistant who was a genetic counselor, performed first hand a thorough ultrasound of the fetus whose chromosomes they had been analyzing over the previous few days. He indicated that an abnormal nuchal fold measurement is usually indicative of Down Syndrome in only 3% of the cases analyzed. A nuchal cyst, however, was a more positive indication of Down Syndrome. He also noted that measurements taken from an untrue angle could result in false readings.

All measurements of the nuchal fold were under 6 mm. No nuchal cyst was present. The lengths of the two thigh bones matched (within measuring error). The specialist was very optimistic that the remainder of the 15 cells analyzed would show no extra copy of the 21st chromosome. Very rarely do they see a "mosaic" where some cells have normal chromosomes and some have the extra 21st chromosome.

His suspicions proved correct. The results of the cell analysis were completed during our visit. No indication of Down

Syndrome was present in any of the 15 cells.

Upon further analysis, he mentioned that the brain was shaped nicely (which would not be the case if spina bifada were present). No evidence of clefting on the lips was found. The stomach looked fine. Both kidneys looked fine. Two umbilical arteries - one on either side of the bladder were noted. After spending such a depressing past few days, this fantastic news was almost impossible to digest.

One last thing that bothered the specialist was that he could not clearly identify the four chambers of the heart. He noticed a discrepancy in the size of the two ventricles. He wasn't sure if there was one large ventricle or two with a very small one next to a large one. If there are two chambers - one bigger than the other, then the chances of a successful repair are higher. Also, the pulmonary artery looked small compared to the aorta.

Although the baby would not roll into a position where he could clearly see the heart, the specialist concluded that a congenital heart defect definitely existed. He immediately asked his assistant to set up an appointment for us at Children's Hospital in town.

Instead of driving home, we found ourselves taking the first of what would turn out to be many trips to Children's. In the past few days our emotions had gone from cautious optimism about the pregnancy, to the depths of depression related to the Down Syndrome news, back to cautious optimism upon news of the misdiagnosis, to a very brief moment of total relief once the misdiagnosis was confirmed, and back to a very scared state not knowing what this congenital heart defect meant for our child's and family's lives.

JUNE, 1997 - WELCOME TO CONGENITAL HEART DISEASE

That same afternoon we were introduced to a cardiologist who would turn out to be the one who would guide us through the upcoming storm. The majority of the next three hours were spent analyzing the heart via an echocardiogram. She said relatively little until she was almost finished. She too was having difficulty getting the fetus in a position where she could clearly see the heart. She also mentioned that the fetus was a bit too young to do an analysis like this.

She suspected that one of three congenital heart diseases existed: Tricuspid Atresia, Tricuspid Atresia with Transposition of the Great Arteries, or Pulmonary Atresia with an Intact Ventricular Septum. She also suggested that we attempt more analysis on another day either fairly soon if we were considering aborting or in two to three weeks otherwise (to give the fetus a chance to develop a bit more).

The issue of abortion quickly transformed from a moral or religious or political debate to a very personal life and death decision. Luckily for us the decision was an easy one. We would move forward with the birth.

The Cardiologist indicated that there was absolutely no danger to my wife and to expect a totally normal pregnancy. She also said to expect about three operations during the child's first three years of life with the first operation occurring within the first two weeks. Amidst all of this medical detail, one of the more baffling aspects was the fact that there was no reason to schedule a c-section. The method of delivery is purely an obstetrics decision. The baby would be in no more or less danger than a child with a normal heart.

Two more echocardiograms were performed over the next three months. Our exposure to and knowledge of heart anatomy and different types of heart defects went from almost nothing to seemingly enough to do the operations ourselves.

Our first tour of the cardiac intensive care unit was a humbling experience. As our legs became weak with the thought of the upcoming challenges that the surroundings seemed to bring to the present, the "routine" activity occurring around the unit made our professions seem so incredibly unimportant. The first sight of the children under such duress created a feeling in your stomach that was never felt before. It was scary to know that the feeling would be even worse when one of those children became our own.

During one of the echocardiogram visits we met the Cardiac Surgeon. Prior to meeting the Surgeon, most of the interaction with medical personnel exuded pessimism. The Surgeon was the first to express optimism. Many statistics were offered to help answer the endless stream of questions that we had.

- Risk of death is about 1% to 2% for the majority of these types of heart conditions.
- Quality of life can essentially be normal with a 95%

probability.

- Single ventricle repairs have been performed for about 20 years.
- 75% of the patients are doing well 15 to 20 years after having undergone this surgery.

Although prenatal diagnosis is about 75% accurate, the Cardiologist concluded accurately that the condition was Pulmonary Atresia with Intact Ventricular Septum. (Refer to Figure 2: Normal Heart, and Figure 3: Heart at Birth.)

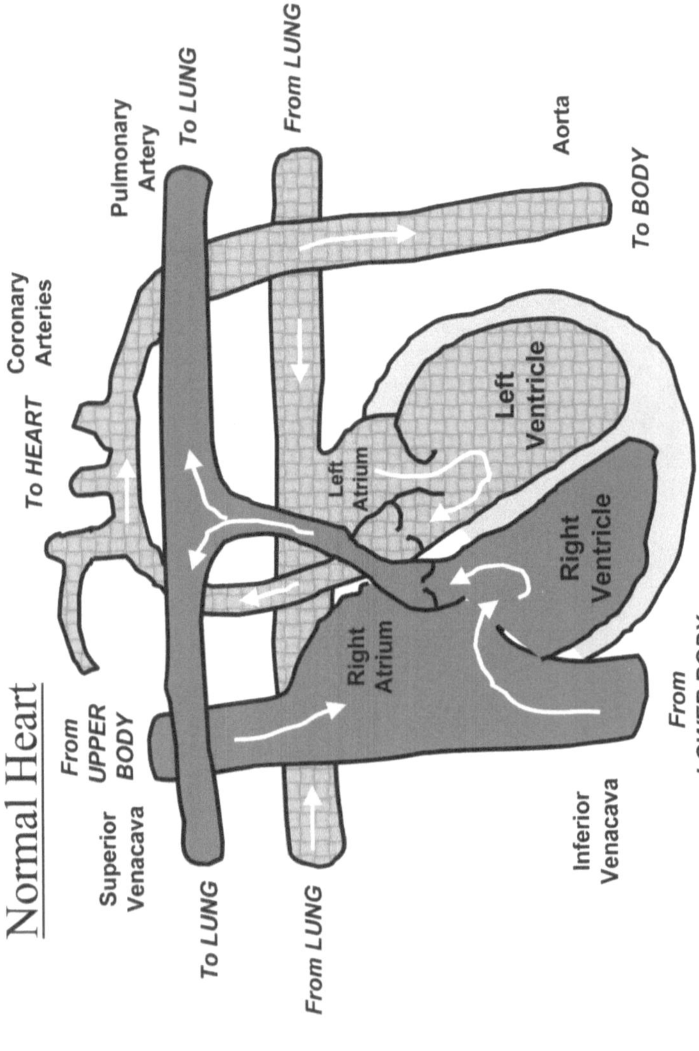

Figure 2: Normal Heart

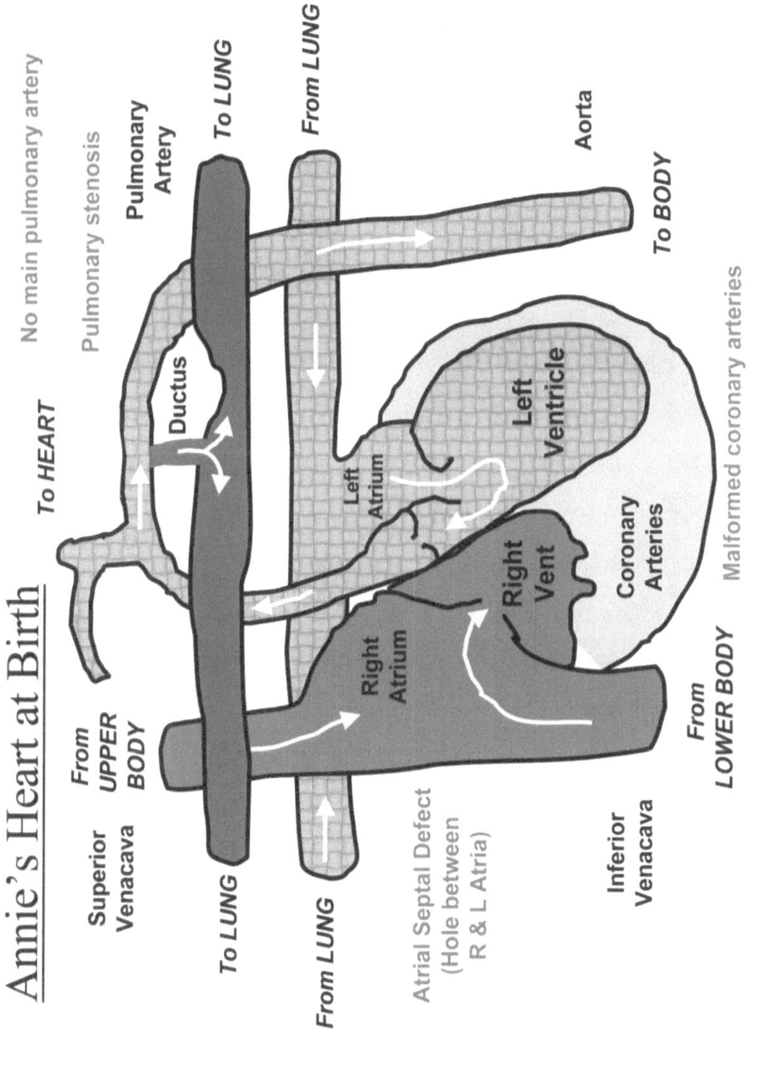

Figure 3: Heart at Birth

NOVEMBER, 1997 - THE BIRTH

Our first lesson in questioning the hospital bureaucracy came on a wasted trip to the birthing Hospital to begin the inducement. Delivery goals were twofold - 1) deliver at the hospital which was about forty-five minutes from our house and 2) increase the chances of delivering when the hospital staff was at its fullest - during the week and during the day. Cervidil gel needed to be applied to soften the cervix for twelve hours prior to starting the Pitossin drip. If the Pitossin drip was scheduled to begin around 8AM on Monday morning and the Cervidil needed to be on for twelve hours prior, it didn't take a medical degree to figure out that someone on the periphery of the situation decided that we should arrive at the hospital ten hours before we really needed to be there. The announcement that we were going home to have one more sunny Sunday afternoon dinner with our family was met with arguments too shallow to keep us in the Hospital for the day.

We arrived back at the Hospital around 7PM. Nobody missed us after all. The unexpected extra time with our son and other relatives was very much appreciated. The Cervidil was applied at 8:10PM. The night was surprisingly restful for us both.

Seventy degrees and sunny on the first day of November was as unusual as what we were about to experience. At 8:15AM the contractions were 3 to 5 minutes apart. The Cervidil was removed and IV started for hydration. By 8:20AM the Pitossin was started followed by an epidural at 9:40AM. At 10AM one of the doctors broke the water. Pushing began at 12:15PM. Annie was born vaginally without incident at 1:50PM at 8 pounds heavy and 20 inches long. The birth of our heart-healthy son three years earlier was much more stressful as his heart rate dipped further and far more frequently than Annie's did during her delivery. Her first gaze at us seemed to last forever. She seemed to be wondering what we were worried about - not that she didn't know what was about to happen but that we didn't know what a fighter she would be.

The priest tried to talk us out of an emergency baptism as someone seemingly must have discussed with him the fact that the situation was not officially considered an emergency. Not taking, "No," for an answer was a decision that left us with one less thing to worry about when things did, in fact, get dire.

Soon Annie was whisked into the portable incubator. She and I and all of our new friends were at the delivery Hospital's Neonatal Intensive Care Unit by 2:05PM. Preparations were made for the long walk through the adjoining hallways to Children's Hospital. By 2:40PM, less than one hour after birth, Annie was plugged into her spot where she would spend the next eighteen days before being transferred to the recovery ward.

NOVEMBER, 1997 - RALLY AROUND THE SHUNT

As Annie was wheeled in the incubator into the Cardiac Intensive Care Unit at Children's Hospital there was much hustle and bustle as the team transferred her from the incubator to a crib and started the Prostaglandin to keep the Ductus from naturally closing and, thus, cutting off the only path for blood to get to Annie's lungs for oxygen. Since Prostaglandin tends to retard the respiratory system, Annie was also intubated so that a ventilator could assist her breathing. The number of tubes and sensors covering Annie's body grew rapidly. The following morning, Annie would head down to the Catheterization Lab to take the first detailed look at her heart in order to devise an appropriate surgical plan.

The catheterization went smoothly on Tuesday morning and by that afternoon, the medical team had reviewed the results. The Cardiac Surgeon sat us down late that afternoon for a very grim conversation. When the most optimistic medical person you have met to date begins a conversation with the fact that "things don't look very good", an indescribable, gut-wrenching feeling rips into your stomach. For the remainder of the discussion, the Surgeon seemed to be talking through us instead of to us. It was as if we weren't in the room with him. Perhaps this was his method of dealing with the delivery of bad news. Perhaps it was his way of preparing himself for a difficult surgery. Either way, the facts were now clear. Annie did indeed have Pulmonary Atresia with an Intact Ventricular Septum. In addition, there was a pinch or "stenosis" in her Pulmonary artery restricting the blood flow to one of her lungs. Finally, her coronary arteries formed in a very unusual manner. Normally there are three main coronary arteries. In Annie's case, she has two medium and many small coronary arteries. This is what really threw the doctors for a loop since it is an extremely rare condition. It remains to be seen whether the structure of her coronary arteries will sufficiently provide the heart with blood.

The goals for surgery on Wednesday morning were to 1) replace the natural Ductus with a Gortex (Blaloc-Taussig) shunt, and 2) repair the pinched artery. (Refer to Figure 4: Blaloc-Taussig (BT) Shunt.) Due to the additional complications, Annie would have to be put on a heart/lung machine adding significantly more risk to the surgery. The Cardiac Surgeon was not sure that Annie would make it through the surgery.

We spent our last moments prior to surgery with her in the surgical prep room feeling nauseous about what would happen next. There was a lot of hustle and bustle as a number of patients were being prepared for surgery. Soon came the time for our final kisses, blessings, and wishes of good luck. Handing Annie to one member of the surgical support team and watching them wheel her crib away to the operating room

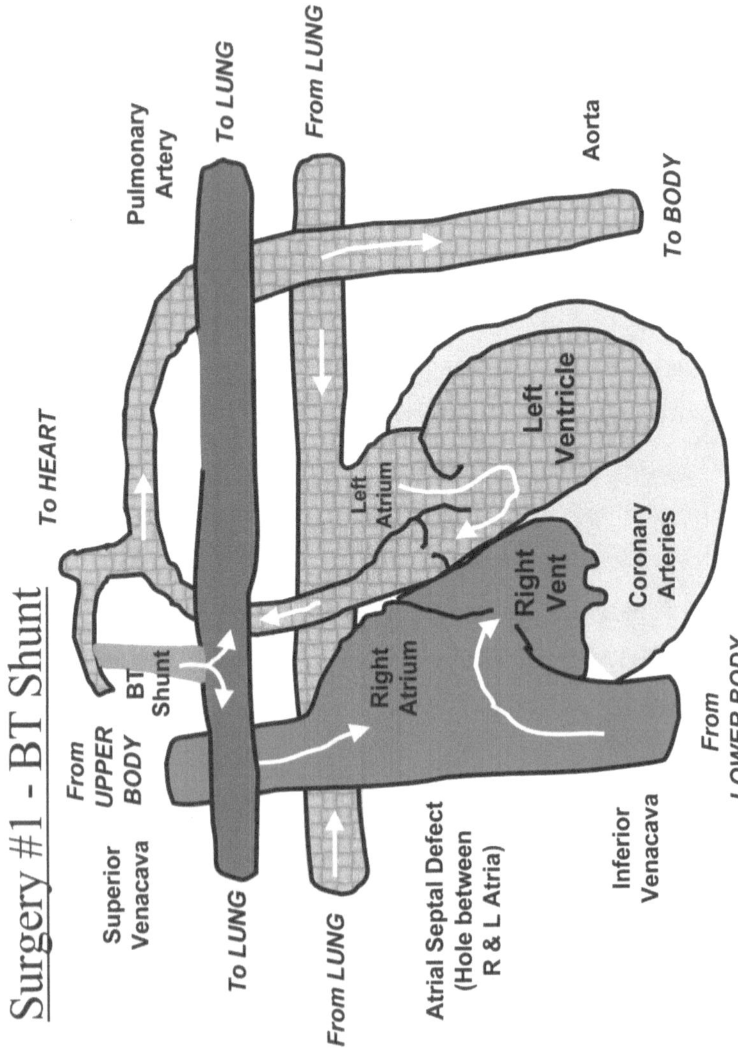

Figure 4: Blaloc-Taussig (BT) Shunt

was one of the most difficult situations any parent would have to face. Time seemed at a standstill for the next few hours as we sweated with anticipation in the waiting room full of anxious families. The anxiety would peak every time the liaison nurse would come out to give progress reports to each of the families. A Hoover Dam's worth of tension broke when we finally received word that Annie had made it through surgery. That unbearable tension would soon shift from one situation, surgery, to the next - recovery.

The night following surgery, we felt enough relief to be able to walk back over to my wife's room at the Birthing Hospital (she had not yet been discharged) for some much-needed rest. Although Annie made it through the night, she apparently had quite a rough time in keeping her blood pressure stable. Her condition stabilized significantly the following day but the pessimism within the medical ranks grew to a demoralizing level. I grew angry with the fact that while everyone seemed to be focused on the negative events, no one other than Annie herself was conscious of the small victories that were progressing her condition forward. She simply kept making slow, steady progress amidst the set-backs that were occurring.

Annie's progress, as small as it was, needed to be magnified a thousand times for all to see in order to drown out the pessimism caused by the many things that were not going well. While contemplating this, I noticed a small whiteboard at each of the patient stations in the Intensive Care Unit. Oddly enough, none of them were being used for anything. It was at this moment in time that "Annie's Rally Board" came to the rescue. On Friday I started a routine where everyday at 5PM, the nurse and I would review all of the positive events of the day and note them on the board near Annie's bedside for all to see. I also began to copy those notes into an electronic mail message that I would send out in the evening to an increasing list of interested supporters all over the world.

The first Rally Board read...

1) The Surgeon got a good night's sleep on Tuesday per orders from mom.
2) Annie survived surgery.
3) Annie's heart is able to pull her out of dips in blood pressure (a reassuring sign that the heart has hope of working on its own.)
4) The kidneys look fine (a sign that she is getting good circulation).
5) P. (She is producing a lot of urine which is key to helping her drain excess fluid that is causing her to be bloated. The chest can't be closed until the swelling subsides.)
6) Poop. (She took a poop yesterday!)
7) The right pulmonary artery was successfully repaired in surgery and is no longer an issue for now.

With each passing day in the Intensive Care Unit the Rally Board updates continued and gained in notoriety. Nurses that weren't even caring for Annie would come by to read The Board. Soon the pessimism was being overshadowed by the continuous display of progress. The growing support that we would receive each morning through email based on the previous day's Rally Board was extremely helpful.

By Monday, Annie's chest was closed as the swelling around the heart had subsided to the point where this was now possible. The importance of this milestone was that no infections developed while waiting for the chest cavity closure. The next day, two chest tubes were removed and she started feeding through a tube to her stomach. On Saturday, a little more than a week after surgery, the ventilator was removed and Annie was breathing on her own. Her first cries since the day she was born sounded better than the most wonderful music one could imagine. Our son met his new sister for the first time that Sunday. Finally, on Thursday, November 20, Annie was kicked out of the Intensive Care Unit for good behavior.

The days on the Recovery Floor were much different than those in the Intensive Care Unit. The nurse-to-patient ratio was much lower since the level of care required was much less than in the ICU. Our involvement in taking care of Annie's basic needs grew rapidly. Our focus dwindled away from the many different levels and types of sustaining drugs to the quantity of formula she was consuming each day. This was the metric that, once exceeded, would be our ticket home.

On Wednesday, November 26, twenty-three days after the birth, we received the best Thanksgiving present anyone could ask for. Annie was discharged from Children's Hospital and sent home for the holiday!

DECEMBER, 1997 - HEART FAILURE OR MILK ALERGY?

Learning how Annie's body functions can be a harrowing experience. She had not been eating well, her weight had not increased in a week or two, and she was vomiting. They admitted her to the Recovery Floor at Children's Hospital on a Wednesday afternoon. At the Hospital her stools tested positive for blood. This was the last straw that set off a wave of tests - blood tests, chest X-Rays, stomach X-Rays, EKG, and an echocardiogram. They were nervous enough to schedule a catheterization on Thursday morning as well. They stopped the oral feeding Wednesday evening. In went the IV line. On went the oxygen tube around her face. She was carted over to the Cardiac ICU at midnight to prepare for Thursday's catheterization.

Annie's Cardiologist thought this might be a good time for us to talk to a representative from the heart transplant team in the event that her heart was failing. This was another gut-wrenching conversation reminiscent of the first presurgery discussion with Annie's Surgeon. It was hard to believe that Annie's journey would lead to a transplant. The option of a heart transplant didn't even hold a strong promise of hope. The thought of going through a heart transplant made what we had just gone through seem trivial.

The catheterization went fine and showed no appreciable difference from the early going. (They did balloon out the area of the Pulmonary artery that was patched. Although this was not really necessary, the fact that they were already in there poking around made it a convenient time to do so.) The echocardiogram looked exactly the same as it had before as did the EKG. The bottom line was that all this testing showed that her problems were not directly related to her heart and were most likely attributable to her diet.

She had been almost exclusively breast feeding. The Pediatrician overreacted to her lack of weight gain and recommended we go back on "Rocket Fuel" (a mix of breast milk, Enfamil powder, and Polycose powder). The apparent mistake was that her diet went from 20-calorie breast milk to 28-calorie Rocket Fuel. Doctors concluded that she could not tolerate such an abrupt change. (She also may have had a cold to further confuse the situation.)

Friday afternoon she went back over to the Recovery Floor and was on straight breast milk (20 calories). Attention was now extremely focused on caloric intake, tracking progress on increasing calories to gain weight while making sure that the rate of increase was slow enough to be tolerable to her system.

I became an expert in formula recipes overnight.

	26 Calorie Mix		28 Calorie Mix		30 Calorie Mix	
Breast Milk (ounces)	Enfamil Powder (teaspoons)	Polycose Powder (teaspoons)	Enfamil Powder (teaspoons)	Polycose Powder (teaspoons)	Enfamil Powder (teaspoons)	Polycose Powder (teaspoons)
1	1/3	1/4	1/3	1/2	1/3	3/4
2	2/3	1/2	2/3	1	2/3	1 1/2
3	1	3/4	1	1 1/2	1	2 1/4
4	1 1/3	1	1 1/3	2	1 1/3	3
5	1 2/3	1 1/4	1 2/3	2 1/2	1 2/3	3 3/4
6	2	1 1/2	2	3	2	4 1/2
7	2 1/3	1 3/4	2 1/3	3 1/2	2 1/3	5 1/4
8	2 2/3	2	2 2/3	4	2 2/3	6
9	3	2 1/4	3	4 1/2	3	6 3/4
10	3 1/3	2 1/2	3 1/3	5	3 1/3	7 1/2
11	3 2/3	2 3/4	3 2/3	5 1/2	3 2/3	8 1/4
12	4	3	4	6	4	9
13	4 1/3	3 1/4	4 1/3	6 1/2	4 1/3	9 3/4
14	4 2/3	3 1/2	4 2/3	7	4 2/3	10 1/2
15	5	3 3/4	5	7 1/2	5	11 1/4
16	5 1/3	4	5 1/3	8	5 1/3	12

Table 1: Rocket Fuel Recipes

Saturday afternoon we slowly cranked her diet up to 22 calories. By Sunday afternoon she was able to tolerate 24 calories. There was no more trace of blood in her stools. Her glucose output was still normal (which is a sign that she was tolerating the changes in caloric content). The oxygen was off while she maintained an oxygen saturation level of 87%.

One more fantastic Holiday present – Annie was discharged and sent home for Christmas on December 23. A raging snowstorm wasn't going to stop us from bringing Annie home. I borrowed a work colleague's four-wheel drive, Sport Utility Vehicle and fought the weather and traffic into the city to bring Mom and Annie home safe and sound.

Even though we were back at home, our Pediatrician remained unsettled with the outcome. Early in January the Pediatrician decided to consult with a Gastrointestinologist. Testing of stool samples indicated an allergy to milk protein. Discussions of heart transplants ceased and were replaced by purchases of Alimentum – a type of formula with a maximum breakdown of proteins. Now we are all able to breathe the next big huge sigh of relief.

FEBRUARY, 1998 - AMBULANCE RIDE FOR A COLD

My first work-related venture away from home was cut short. I received word that Annie was taken to the emergency room of the local hospital due to low oxygen levels. Officially, she contracted a case of Bronchiolitis. . The congestion in her lungs had caused the levels of oxygen in her blood (O_2 saturation) to go down enough that she needed to be in the hospital and put on oxygen.

Rushing home as fast as I could, I met my whole family at the local hospital. It was a very long and painful ride home for me as I contemplated the many different scenarios that could occur. The local Hospital Staff were not permitted to let us make the forty-minute drive downtown to Children's Hospital ourselves so, instead, we waited for three hours in the emergency ward for the transport team to arrive. After what seemed like an eternity, the ambulance finally showed up and rushed us to Children's Hospital. Cars were frantically trying to get out of our way as the sirens blared at the intersections. Two cars collided as the first driver's last second indecision caused another driver to plow into him. Thankfully, no one appeared to be injured. It was very ironic that we were being rushed to the Hospital after such a long wait. Nevertheless, I have to admit that Annie and

I had fun on the unusual and adventurous ride.

Although her eating had slowed down quite a bit just prior to her arrival in the Hospital, it had picked back up after being on oxygen for just one day. On the second day of her stay Annie broke her all-time eating record. She still couldn't seem to shake the oxygen, however. Her lungs needed more time to clear up. I was nervous that if her lungs didn't clear up enough to go home in a day or two that we could be staying there for the week if she were to pick up the funk that her roommate had. I figured that by the time she got discharged that I was going to be admitted. As it turned out, Annie didn't pick up the funk but it still took six days to get back on track and discharged.

For the first time, there were no holidays to go home to. But it was still just as good to be home.

MAY, 1998 - ANOTHER GLENN SKY ROCKETS TO SUCCESS

On April 29 we had just gotten back from Children's Hospital. Annie had a catheterization the previous morning and an echocardiogram that morning. Although it was the usual agony of putting in IV lines and drawing blood after the catheterization, the outcome was good. No new news was good news. The pressures in the arteries looked nice and low. No problem vessels had sprouted. All systems were go for the Glenn operation on May 12 (assuming we didn't get bumped by a heart transplant patient).

SURGICAL DETAILS

There were two tasks planned for surgery this morning:

TASK 1: Bi-directional Glenn

Since Annie was born with no blood flow to her lungs (pulmonary atresia = very small right atria and no main pulmonary artery), she underwent surgery on the third day of her life to install a Gortex tube (Blaloc-Taussig shunt) between her aorta (through which oxygenated red blood is pumped out to the body) and her pulmonary artery (through which blue blood is pumped to the lungs for more oxygen). This configuration is what allowed Annie to survive her first 6 months of life. The left ventricle not only does its usual job of pushing blood out to the body but it also has to push blood to the lungs. This adds stress to the heart but is the only way to get patients with this condition through early life until pressure in the lungs drops to levels low enough to perform the Glenn operation.

The Bi-directional Glenn consists of

a) removing the Gortex shunt,
b) detaching the superior vena cava (the vessel that delivers blue blood from the upper extremities to the right atria) from the heart,
c) reconnecting the superior vena cava to the pulmonary artery at the point where the shunt used to be attached.

(Refer to Figure 5: Bidirectional Glenn.)

With this new configuration, half of the blue blood returning to the heart to get pumped to the lungs for oxygen now simply flows by gravity around the heart and directly into the lungs. As a result, the volume of blood going through the left ventricle is significantly reduced which, in turn, reduces the stress on the heart. The heart shrinks a bit and pumps more strongly. This configuration is considered to be "bi-directional" since the blue blood flowing from the superior vena cava now flows down both the right and left pulmonary arteries (going to the right and left lung respectively).

A few years from now, the second half of the blue blood returning to the heart (through the inferior vena cava from the lower extremities) to get pumped to the lungs gets rerouted

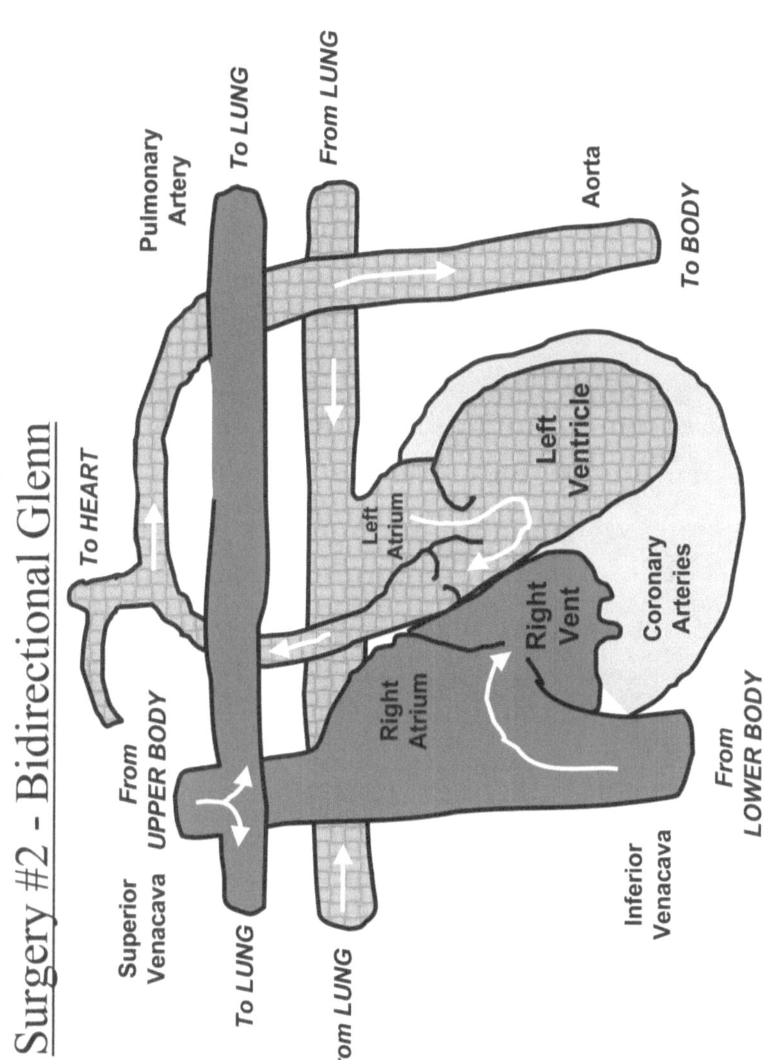

Figure 5: Bidirectional Glenn

around the heart. This final configuration is called the Fontan.

TASK 2: Pulmonary Artery repair

Annie was also born with pulmonary arterial stenosis. (No offense to those of you in the medical profession but we all know that doctors, like lawyers, use very complicated terminology to describe very simple things in order to confuse the rest of us so that they can make more money.) This is simply a pinched section of the artery leading to the lungs. This "pinch" was repaired during the initial surgery and ballooned out a month later during an exploratory catheterization. The Surgeon had planned on using some of the pericardium (tissue around the outer part of the heart) to enlarge this repaired section of the artery. During today's surgery, however, he decided that this was not necessary since the artery looked better than he had expected.

TUESDAY'S RALLY BOARD (5/12/98)

- Annie's Surgeon followed mom's orders again and got a good night's sleep.
- Annie did very well in surgery.
- Pulmonary Artery repair was not needed.
- Intermittent Mechanical Ventilation weaned from 24 to 20 breaths per minute.
- Annie was awake and moving by 1PM!!!

Annie was put on the heart/lung machine during surgery. She went on and came off of it well.

Current medications are:

Dopamine (6 micrograms/kilo/minute) - blood pressure support.

Fentanyl (5 micrograms/kilo/hour) - pain medication that is much stronger than morphine

She had a bad reaction to the combination of morphine (pain) and versed (sedative) this afternoon around 2PM. Her blood pressure dropped to a dangerously low level. They quickly were able to stabilize her. After this episode, they replaced the morphine/versed combo with fentanyl.

Intubated (breathing tube affixed) with 60% oxygen starting at 24 breaths per minute.

Oxygen saturation is fluctuating from high 80s to high 70s.

One chest tube. The chest is closed during the operation so we don't have to wait a few days like we did the last time for the chest to be closed in the ICU.

By the way, the nurse that took such good care of Annie and us the last time, took care of Annie today in the ICU. Even though she did her usual great job, I can't really make mention of it here since she is now on the email list and we don't want it going to her head until after Annie is out of the ICU.

WEDNESDAY'S RALLY BOARD (5/13/98)

Another very good day.

- Extubated!

The ventilator was removed this afternoon. This is a tube that goes up her nasal passage into her trachea. It took about 10 or 12 days to get to this point the last time.

- Attempted to feed.

Took a little bit of sugar water.

- Dopamine (blood pressure med) dropped from 4 micrograms/kilogram/minute to 3.
- Removed peripheral IV from the right hand.
- Started sucking her fingers.
- One common atrial line pulled.

I misstated yesterday the fact that she only has one chest tube to drain fluid from the chest cavity. She actually started with 3. One of the three was removed this afternoon.

- Moved to a brand new bed.

Annie is now in a crib which is yet another step towards heading to the Recovery Floor.

- Gas mania

Achieved Harvard textbook Arterial Blood Gas (ABG) of 7.41 pH, 40 PCO2 (carbon dioxide), 40 PO2 (oxygen). This is the exact mix of gases that are supposed to be in the blood.

- P

Urine output is always a good thing since the patient takes on fluid during surgery. Annie is running 100 cc's negative which means she put out 100 cc's more than she took in today.

THURSDAY'S RALLY BOARD (5/14/98)

The ICU lost a 2-month old baby on Tuesday night a few spaces down from Annie - a major wake-up call for us all. An eerie calm fell upon the entire floor. We now know that an empty bed space doesn't always mean good things. As bad as we thought we had it, we had no right, comparatively speaking, to feel sorry for ourselves. In fact, we are feeling very lucky to be where we are right now!

- Another good day for Annie.
- All chest tubes are history.
- Bottle feeding.

Started late last night by devouring a 4-oz bottle.

- No more Dopamine.
- Arterial Line is history.

This is a line in the groin area used for continuous blood pressure measurements as well as occasional blood gas checks.

- Foley Disconnected.

Back to filling up diapers instead of bags.

- Mom held Annie for a bit so she could get a peek at the Major League Baseball Park out of her window.

FRIDAY'S RALLY BOARD (5/15/98)

- RECOVERY FLOOR!!!

They kicked Annie out of the Intensive Care Unit today for good behavior. She's now in the on-deck circle to get booted out of the hospital - sixth floor of the east wing. If she continues on her current pace, then I would guess she will get discharged sometime between Sunday and Tuesday. She is eating and sleeping well. She only has one IV line left in her foot and a pacing wire that is nestled next to the bottom of her heart. (The pacing wire doesn't get pulled until right before she goes home. They keep it in as a precaution in case they need to give the heart some electrical stimulus in the event of an emergency.)

Dad is on solo hospital duty this weekend. Mom is headed south on Saturday to pick our son up from his cousin's house and to assess the physical damage the two 4-year-olds inflicted on my sister and brother-in-law's house this past week. They will be back home on Sunday night.

Annie is in a luxurious single but she lost her window along with the view of the ballpark. If you call and we don't answer, it's probably because we are cranking tunes. (We can get away with quite a bit when mom's not around.) There isn't much of a selection on the jukebox downstairs near the stage. But they do have a copy of Marvin Gaye singing, "I Heard It Through the Grapevine". I hold Annie in my arms and we dance alone on the stage while we (ok, "I") sing along. I'm so happy to be able to do this that I start getting choked up and can't finish singing the song.

SUNDAY (5/17/98)

We can still feel the stress of last Sunday. I can still hear our priest giving Annie one last blessing before surgery wondering if we would be back for more. If you would have asked us then what we would be doing this Sunday, there seemingly were only two answers - 1) rocking grooves in the floor of the Intensive Care Unit or 2) grieving. To think that we would be home, that Annie would be on one less medication than she was the past

6 months, that she would be eating more than she did a week ago, and that the diapers would be getting filled up so much that one would think there were two people contributing, were thoughts that didn't even make it to the "Yeah, right. I don't think so" column.

I felt so lucky and blessed to be walking out of the hospital today with our daughter. I thought about those parents that started last week in the same position as we did but ended it much differently and wondered what we had done to deserve our fate. I knew that our prayers were answered. Don't take the simple things in life for granted. Focus on the positive. Keep the faith.

MARCH, 1999 – POST GLENN CATH

It has been a very rough and stressful two days but Annie is finally resting comfortably. In the words of her Cardiologist, "The cath went perfectly".

Yesterday they put an IV in her left hand and did a lung scan, blood test, chest X-ray, and urine sample. The IV went in the first shot (which was a pleasant surprise) thanks to the nurse from the Cath Lab (i.e., expert at IV insertion) who just happened to be in the Nuclear Medicine area when we arrived for the lung scan. They inject some sort of radioactive fluid into the IV for the lung scan which measures the amount of blood flow into each lung. Her left lung was only getting about 20% blood flow due to the narrowing in her main pulmonary artery.

There was talk last night about possibly inserting a stent (steel cage) in the area of the narrowing. There was also talk about having to block off collateral arteries stemming from the aorta to the lungs. (If the blood flow from the collateral arteries carrying oxygenated blood is too high, then it retards the flow of venus blood which is supposed to be going back to the lungs for more oxygen.)

As it turned out, a ballooning of the narrow artery was sufficient (no stent needed) and the blood flow from the collateral arteries to the lungs was deemed insignificant.

Soon after Annie was back from the recovery area she was sucking down a Citrus Burst fruit smoothie from Jera Juice.

They did a follow-up lung scan this afternoon to measure the increase in blood flow to the left lung. We are awaiting the results of that. The doctor that assisted in the catheterization showed us the images that were taken before and after the ballooning. The difference in blood flow to the top portion of the left lung was amazing.

More pain and agony on the second night. Just when we thought we were done after the lung scan, we went back for an x-ray. They also needed to draw blood and couldn't get it out of her IV line. After one last round (hopefully) of needle sticking, Annie fell fast asleep after another long, hard day at the Hospital.

If all continues to go well, then we should be going home at some point tomorrow.

WEDNESDAY (3/3/99)

Annie was discharged right before noon. All is well.

APRIL, 2000 – PRE-FONTAN CATH

A year has passed. Annie is doing very well. Her blood saturation level is in the mid 80's. She has hit the weight charts and is riding the lower percentiles for her age. Although she gets winded, she is very active and keeps up with the best of them. It feels like another surgery is just not worth it. But the doctors assure us that the long-term effects of the Fontan (refer to Figure 6: The Fontan) will work in Annie's favor as she gets older.

WHY DO THE FONTAN?

The doctors don't expect an outwardly noticeable difference in Annie after the Fontan. There are two reasons why the Fontan is performed: 1) patients that are left with a Glenn configuration form tiny connections between the arteries and veins in their lungs [pulmonary arterial venous malformations (AVM)] that prevent blood from reaching the capillaries. Pulmonary AVM leaves the patient cyanotic and extra blood is sent to the heart which is not good. 2) the Fontan configuration gets the liver back into the lung side of the circulation which studies have found to have positive effects.

POST FONTAN ISSUES

After the Fontan, patients are usually left with a small tunnel between the right and left side of the heart (called a

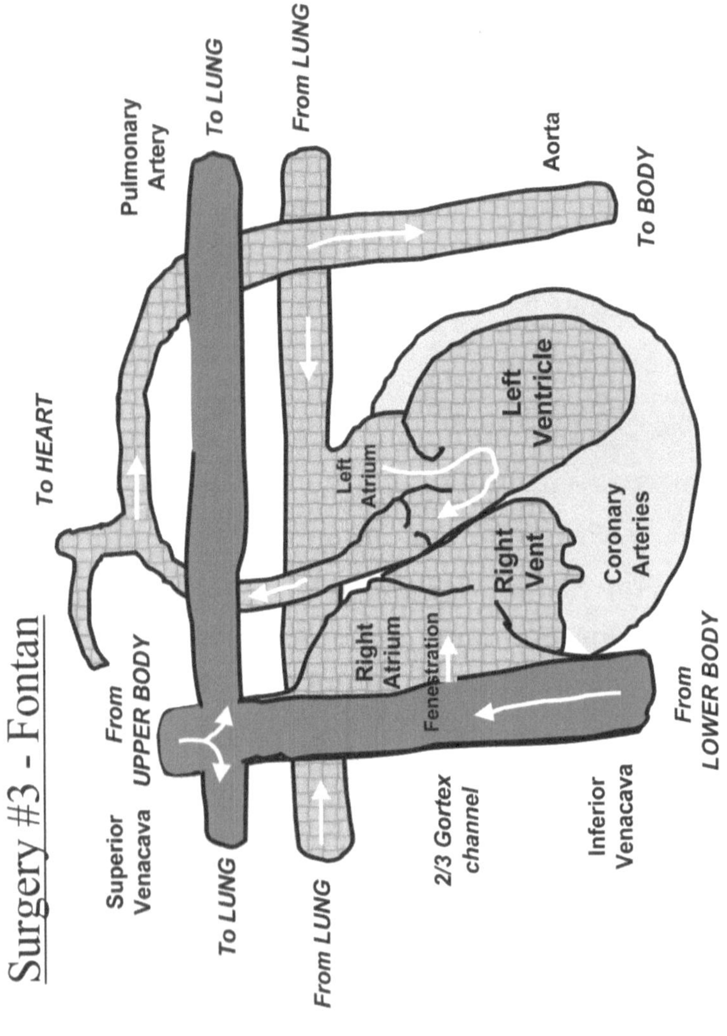

Figure 6: The Fontan

fenestration). The medical community debates whether the fenestration should be left open or closed. (The Head of Cardiology at the Hospital invented a device called The Star Flex which is designed to close the tunnel. It is installed using a catheter.)

If the fenestration is closed, then the patient's saturation levels go up (which is believed to be good) but the patient is more susceptible to an air bubble causing a stroke. If the fenestration is left open, more blood can get through the heart (via the left side) in the event that there is a downstream blockage (like that which would be caused by pneumonia clogging up circulation in the lungs). As a result, the patient can better fight pneumonia. Annie's doctors advocate leaving it open.

TUESDAY (4/25/00)

The bad news is that we just finished 2 rough days in the hospital to collect data for Annie's upcoming surgery in May. The good news is that 1) the results were much better than expected and 2) we all got to sleep in our beds at home both nights!

Monday - In at 8:30AM. Height, weight, blood pressure, EKG, chest X-Ray all were pretty easy. The lung scan is nasty since they have to stick her with a needle to inject radioactive isotopes to check the blood flow to each lung. (The results were nearly normal on both sides!) At least that was the extent of the nastiness for the day. Annie was not happy to say the least. They were able to simultaneously draw enough blood for her blood work saving her a second stick.

We had to stick around until 2:30PM so that 14 doctors could listen to her lungs to make sure last week's cough wouldn't be an issue for the catheterization. Each agreed that there was no issue.

Tuesday - We were on the schedule to be one of the first cases in the cath lab at 7:15AM. They called the night before to tell us that we got bumped to 2nd case due to an emergency. 2nd case goes in around 10:30AM. We showed up at the hospital at 10AM. No solid food 8 hours ahead of time and no clear liquids 2 hours prior. We kept getting bumped back and didn't go into the lab until 3PM. Annie was quite a trooper having had only 2 bites of jello and some apple juice all day.

The medication that they gave her to put her out was supposed to take effect in 10 minutes. 35 minutes later she was still watching Barney. That meant we had to take her into the cath lab awake and put in the IV. This was the worst part of both days by far.

She was out of the lab in 2 hours - 5PM. Pressures were perfect for the Fontan operation. The pinch in her pulmonary artery is almost undetectable at this point. The surgically repaired area has grown up with her! Coronary arteries are functioning well.

She was not happy to be in a room on the Recovery Floor.

But by 8PM she had downed a few cups of juice and started in on the fish crackers. She recovered quickly enough that they discharged us at 10PM. She's sleeping soundly in her own bed.

MAY, 2000 – THE FONTAN

TUESDAY (5/23/00)

Pre-op tests went well today. Annie is cleared for surgery and so far we have not gotten bumped.

She gets one more night's sleep in her own bed. We will be in the hospital at 7:30AM. They will start around 8:30AM. Surgery should go about 3 or 4 hours. We won't be reunited with her in the ICU until about 1:30PM. They probably won't let her wake up for about 24 hours.

WEDNESDAY (5/24/00)

We arrived at the hospital bright and early. After checking in, we made our way to the surgery preparation area. The room was bustling with activity as teams of medical staff went about their preparations. I have never been so nervous in my life. The stress of the situation was unbearable. If ever I was going to have a heart attack it would be now. (Looking on the bright side, there would be no better place to have one.) I paced anxiously as we waited along with 3 or 4 people on the surgical team for the mind-numbing drugs to take affect so that they could take Annie into the operating room and start an IV. Annie's angel doll that went with her during the first two surgeries seemed ready for her biggest challenge yet. The previous surgeries seemed so much easier as this time Annie was old enough to sense that something bad was happening.

Then came the moment. My wife and I each kissed Annie wondering if it would be the last. As they carried her away, our hearts seemed to rip out of our chests and follow Annie into the operating room. Our eyes quickly welled up with tears. It was much harder to hand over a young child to the surgical team than it was to hand over an infant. We had two-plus years with Annie – watching her come to life and develop her personality. The power of the moment's emotions resulted in a physically weakening feeling. My body felt completely drained of energy. I honestly wasn't sure if I would make it through the surgery, regardless of Annie's fate. The next four hours would seem like four years.

Surgery began around 8:45AM as scheduled. We went to the unfortunately familiar waiting area and took our positions amongst the other nervous parents and relatives. I'm not sure how quickly I was spinning the rosary but the Hail Mary's were flying by fast and furiously.

As time dragged on, the liaison nurse began her nerve-racking duty of providing each family with surgical updates. Each time she approached us, we held our breaths until she got past that great first sentence of, "Everything is going well." Our prayers were answered as we heard that sentence each and every time. The last update came directly from the Surgeon who greeted us with a smile and great news as he escorted us into a nearby discussion room. After hearing the details of how all went well, one wonders what to say or do to the person that just reconstructed your daughter's heart and gave her a new lease on life. The conversation ends with a stunned but joyous, "Thank you", and handshake.

Surgery wrapped up around 12:30PM. Wow! The weight of the world was off of our shoulders – at least temporarily. Walking out of the waiting room, we felt elated, exhausted, anxious, and concerned, all at the same time.

Goals for the afternoon were to

1) make sure that there is no clotting in the hole (fenestration) to the right atrium
2) make sure that there is no excessive post-operative bleeding.

WEDNESDAY'S RALLY BOARD (5/24/00)

- Annie made it through surgery with flying colors!!!
- She went onto and came off of the heart/lung machine with no issues.
- She was awake and shaking her head in response to questions by mid afternoon.
- Chest tubes are draining at 20 to 30 cc/hour
- Kicking feet and arms. (She had to be tied down.)
- Dopamine is at 7.5
- Ventilator is down to 12 from 16 breaths per minute.
- No signs of fenestration clotting.
- Got a blessing from our Church's Deacon.

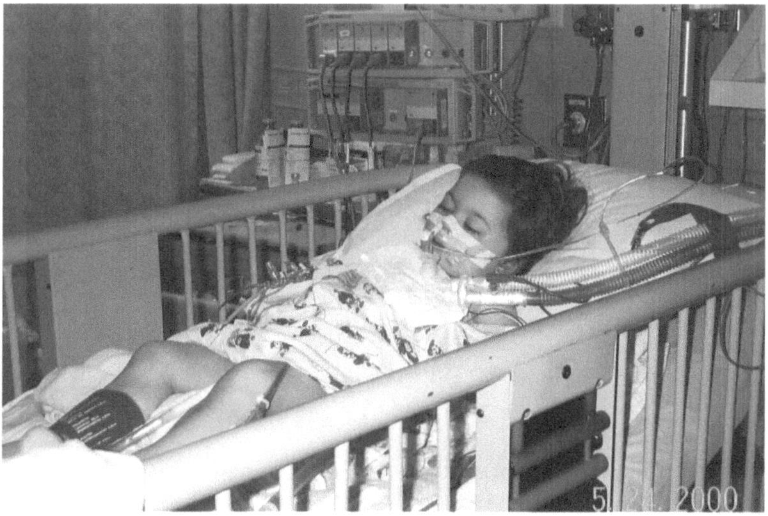

Figure 7: Shortly after Fontan Surgery

THURSDAY'S RALLY BOARD (5/25/00)

Recovery is going well. Medically, it was a delightfully uneventful day!

- Annie is breathing on her own. (Extubated last night at 9PM.)
- Dopamine is down to 3 mics/kilo/min
- Blood pressure has stabilized to the 75 to 80 range.
- Oxygen saturation has been in the high 70's to low 80's.
- Cooling blanket has been removed as she has fought off the post-op fever.
- Had a popsicle last night.
- Drinking apple juice (since they ran out of beer).
- Watching Barney (we were all going through

withdrawal until then).
- Reading books.
- Tie downs have been removed so she can resume sucking her favorite fingers and continue her attempts at removing her belly button.

They started Milrenome last night - a drug that helps open up her capillaries to help blood flow to the extremities.

The newborn baby in the space next to Annie's was airlifted here a week ago from Alabama. She had heart failure and was put on an extra-corporeal membrane oxygenation (ECMO) machine which is an external machine that takes the place of the heart. One can only survive in this mode for about 2 weeks. She needed a heart transplant. The wait for a new heart can be 9 months to a year if you are lucky. The baby's future was obviously doomed.

Yesterday, a heart became available and was flown in from Philly. The baby had a heart transplant last night and is doing fine.

It's very hard to describe the emotions that this brings out in us. Often we are surrounded by things that aren't right in the world. But when something goes so incredibly right, you feel like running down the hall, sticking your head out the window, and screaming so loud that everyone on the street below can't help but stop what their doing and pay attention for a second.

I can't even begin to imagine how the child's parents feel.

FRIDAY'S RALLY BOARD (5/26/00)

- Chest tube drainage is slowing. (Plural tubes are down to about 10 cc/hr; Media Stinal down to <1 cc/hr.)
- Dopamine is off.
- Milrinone is off.
- Blood pressure is in the 90s (with some help from an external pace maker). (90 to 100 is normal for her.)
- Oxygen through a nasal canula down to 1/2 liters/min from 2 liters/min at the start of the day.
- Oxygen saturation has been in the mid 80's.
- Platelet count has stabilized.
- No more blood given today.
- Left atrial line removed (the catheter into the left atrium).
- Atrial line for taking blood gases removed.
- Neck IV removed.
- Foley catheter removed.
- Eating crackers, Cheerios, and a popsicle.
- We thwarted an Annie escape attempt from her crib.

SATURDAY'S RALLY BOARD (5/27/00)

- Removed a chest tube this morning (Medial Stinal).
- Shut off oxygen and removed nasal tube.
- Shut off IV fluids.
- Started taking Lasix orally.
- Sat up for most of the day on either mom's or dad's lap.
- Did some painting.
- External pace maker reduced from 138 bpm to 124.

Annie's nurse today happens to be our neighbor. Annie is getting well enough that people are starting to wonder why she is still in the ICU. Her biggest hurdle to leaving is the pace maker. It is very typical after a Fontan that, due to swelling in the heart, pacing is required. She won't move out of the ICU until her heart can keep the pace unassisted or a tiny pacemaker is installed to do it for her.

SUNDAY'S RALLY BOARD (5/28/00)

- Lungs clear
- Blood pressure at 91 (sleeping)
- Oxygen saturation in mid 80s.
- Stood up and walked around.
- Plural chest tubes' output down to 55 cc's today from 115 yesterday.
- Pacer down to 120 bpm.
- Dad only had to watch Inspector Gadget twice.

They were considering turning the pacer off for about an hour today to see how she would do but postponed until tomorrow. She was not able to keep either breakfast or lunch down. (Dad got breakfast. Mom got lunch.) She was back to her happy self by dinner and ate well. There is an outside chance that the last of the chest tubes will be pulled tomorrow.

MONDAY'S RALLY BOARD (5/29/00)

- Blood work results were excellent. (She had to get stuck to get blood drawn but they used a topical numbing drug, Emla, which worked wonders! Why don't they use this all the time?)
- Yesterday's chest tube output turned out to be 100 cc's. Today she is down to 80. Output slowed considerably. There were 3 hours in a row today where the output was zero. Let's hope for the best tomorrow in getting these boat anchors pulled.
- 3 good meals today - all kept down. Dinner was especially good as Aunt, Uncle, and cousins brought us in a home-barbecued chicken dinner to celebrate Memorial Day.
- IV fluids were turned down from 45 cc/hr to 25 while she took in 240 cc's orally (none of which was beer).
- Poop!
- And last but not least (pay no attention to the order in which these are listed), our favorite nurse was taking as good care of Annie today as she did through the initial surgeries.

TUESDAY'S RALLY BOARD (5/30/00)

Very rough day but ended on a high note. What a rollercoaster!

- Shut off the pacing tonight! Heart rate held in the high 80s to low 90s. Blood pressure stayed in the 90s. The sinus node is still not firing. She is going to ride the night on her own as long as the numbers stay solid.

(The sinus node at the top of the atrium should send out an electrical impulse first causing the upper chamber to contract. Next, the AV node at the junction of the atrium and ventricle should fire next causing the ventricle to contract. This is called a "sinus rhythm". If the upper node does not fire but the bottom one does, then the upper chamber is drained of blood as opposed to pushing out the blood. This is called a "junctional rhythm". The heart rate slows as a result and this method of pumping is not as efficient. Nevertheless, one can survive with such a situation. Once the swelling in the atrium subsides, it is very common that the firing of the sinus node resumes.)

- Fought off a temperature of 104.
- Chest tube output is continuing to slow. Down to a total of 50 cc's versus 80 at the same time yesterday. They split the remaining tubes in two tonight and might pull one tomorrow once they determine which one may have stopped putting out fluid. Started some general antibiotics (genimycin and vancomycin) in response to the fever. Blood tests for infection won't be completed for another 48 hours. Antibiotics will be stopped at that time if they find nothing or changed to something more specific once they determine what the bacteria reacts most negatively to.

WEDNESDAY'S RALLY BOARD (5/31/00)

There's only one other Rally Board better than this one...

- Kicked out of the ICU for good behavior!
- The last of the chest tubes removed this afternoon.
- Fever is down to 101/102.
- Initial results on blood test show no signs of infection. More results tomorrow.
- Blood pressure, pulse rate, and oxygen saturation holding steady even though we are still in a junctional rhythm.
- Took a walk from our new room to the play room!

A simple walk down the hall never felt so good. It's something that we all take for granted every day. But this walk was different. We might as well have been walking on the moon because that was the significance that was being felt.

THURSDAY'S RALLY BOARD (6/1/00)

- Echocardiogram looked good. No signs of fluid around the heart.
- Still no signs of infection from the blood analysis.
- Temperature down to 100.
- Saw some brief signs of a sinus rhythm last night.
- White cell count going down which is another sign that there is no significant infection driving the fever.

The biggest remaining issue between us and home right now is this fever. They are being extra conservative to check all possible signs of infection.

FRIDAY'S RALLY BOARD (6/2/00)

- White blood cell count holding steady.
- Final report on blood cultures says no infection.
- One more day of antibiotics.
- Fever just under 100 now.
- Pacing wires pulled.

SATURDAY'S RALLY BOARD (6/3/00)

- Got outside for a few hours this afternoon. They were having "Kids' Day" in the courtyard.
- Fever holding steady.
- Last day of antibiotics.
- Got our hair done.
- Did some dancing with daddy.

The main issue right now is some fluid around the lungs. Lasix should take care of this.

SUNDAY'S RALLY BOARD (6/4/00)

- The first non-needle day I can remember in awhile.
- Antibiotics stopped.
- Temperature gone.
- P-waves are back tonight.
- Ate well and kept it all down.

They are really running out of reasons to keep us around now. We're down to some fluid around the lungs. There was a slight increase on Friday. The danger is that the fluid continues to increase and they make us stick around until the Lasix makes it go away. Tomorrow morning's x-ray will tell us how we are doing on that front.

TUESDAY'S RALLY BOARD (6/6/00)

- People are beginning to wonder why we are here.
- Annie walked the long way from the main lobby to 6 East (using the elevators, of course).
- White blood cell count remains the same as the past 2 days.
- Drank 18.6 ounces of fluids today.
- The switch from Lasix to Diuril went smoothly. (They switched to Diuril, another type of diuretic, to test a theory that she may have developed an allergic reaction to Lasix.)

Annie's temp started at 102 today, came down to 100, and ended up at 103. Nevertheless, she has been very active, happy, hungry, and thirsty. The only rational theory is that the effusion around the lungs is causing the fever. X-ray tomorrow AM will tell us how the effusion is doing.

My patience with the situation is wearing thin. Will the see-sawing temperatures ever end?

THURSDAY'S RALLY BOARD (6/8/00)

- Lung effusion (fluid in the sack surrounding the lung) is gone.
- Blood tests continue to show no sign of infection but point to an inflammation instead.

- It looks like the cause of the temperature was identified.

An effusion in the heart has formed behind the atrium. This is very common and is treated with Motrin. Even though Annie still has a fever, they almost let us go today. I say, "almost", because her potassium level is too low since we did such a good job peeing off the lung effusion. (Potassium is passed out through urine.)

After having a strategy session with the Charge Nurse, we are armed with our special potassium-enhanced lemonade as well as a banana/orange juice smoothie this afternoon. If her blood shows an acceptable level of potassium tomorrow morning, we will have our walking papers. Let's hope for the best.

FRIDAY'S RALLY BOARD (6/9/00)

The Long-awaited Rally Board...

- We're home!

Annie ate enough bananas and drank enough potassium supplement to make it over the 4.0 potassium threshold in her blood analysis today. We received our walking papers late this morning and were home by 2PM. She will be on Diuril (diuretic to make sure the effusion in the lung doesn't come back - i.e., keep the internal fluid levels down) once a day for about 2 weeks. She is also taking Motrin 3 times a day to make sure the inflammation in the heart goes away and stays away so that the effusion behind the heart dissipates. We will go back on Monday at 3PM for another echocardiogram, chest x-ray, and ekg. She may come off the Motrin at that point. She will also be taking an aspirin a day for the rest of her life to help minimize the risk of clotting.

Seventeen days ago we weren't sure if we would ever see this day. We're thankful for everyone's prayers and support. The prayers were answered - big time! One thing I can say for sure. It will be a long time before I will ever watch the movies, "Inspector Gadget", "Mighty Joe Young", " Iron Giant", or "Barney".

It is difficult to describe the feeling of walking out of the hospital with a child that went through what Annie did and have her looking so good and being so happy. It was a very emotional step to place a foot on the outside sidewalk with Annie in my arms – a monumental step in the right direction. Once again… Don't take the simple things in life for granted. Focus on the positive. Keep the faith.

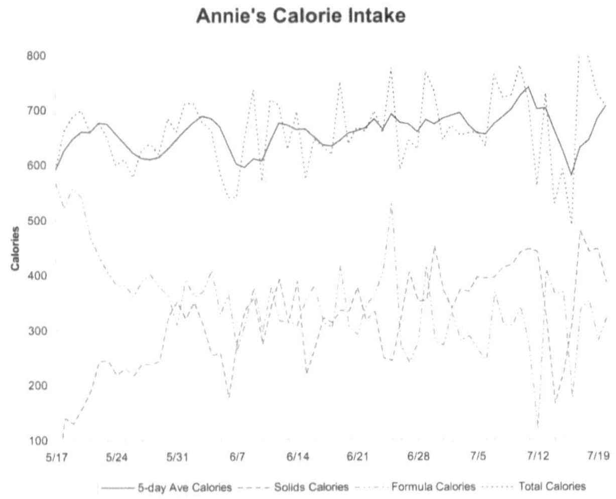

Figure 8: Caloric Intake Before, During, and After Fontan

OCTOBER, 2002 – POST-FONTAN CATH

It has been nearly two and a half years since Annie's Fontan surgery. She has gone back to the Hospital for major check-ups every six months or so. She has done amazingly well. Four years ago who would have ever imagined that she would be in the twenty-fifth percentile of height and weight, going to school, taking dance classes, swimming, playing tennis, and skiing!

Although this catheterization is technically elective, it is being highly recommended by Annie's doctors. There are three goals for the procedure:

1.) Close the fenestration - the hole intentionally left from the Fontan surgery between the right and left sides of the heart.

The doctors now feel that the benefits of closing the fenestration (increasing the percentage of oxygen in the blood to more normal levels and blocking a potential passageway for a blood clot reaching the brain) outweigh the risks of closing it (closing a pressure relief path in the event of a pressure build-up in the lungs as would happen during pneumonia).

2.) Perform electrical tests to help in the decision to implant a pacemaker or not and, in the event that the decision is to go ahead with the pacemaker, to formulate a plan for the type of pacemaker to use and where to install it.

Annie's heart continues to function electrically in a

"junctional" rhythm (no electrical impulse causing contraction of the Atrium or upper chamber) as opposed to a "sinus" rhythm (electrical impulse causes the Atrium to contract following by a second impulse at the junction of the Atrium and Ventricle causing the bottom chamber to contract). Although this is normal immediately following the Fontan surgery, most patients transition from a junctional rhythm to a normal sinus rhythm shortly after surgery. Annie's heart never made the transition. Doctors speculate that it is not good for the heart to function in a junctional rhythm for the life of a patient.

3.) Evaluate the state of the coronary arteries.

Annie's coronary arteries were formed in a very abnormal way. Doctors don't really understand the long-term effects of such a condition and continue to monitor the situation.

PRE-CATH WORK-UP

The doctor's travel schedule bumped us from our original October 4 work-up day to Friday, October 19. The night before, we told Annie that we had to visit the Cardiologist in the morning and that there would be one ouchie (drawing blood for blood analysis). She melted into tears. But, in line with the roller coaster ride that comes with medical challenges, she quickly recovered. Our discussion turned to making fun of certain close relatives who have a habit of snoring loudly. We were laughing so much that Annie had to abruptly end the conversation to announce that her "cheeks hurt from smiling too much" which, of course, caused further pain after we burst out in laughter again.

The work-up day went well. It started with having one of Annie's favorite Recovery Floor nurses from the Fontan recovery as our liaison for the day. We started with an easy echocardiogram, followed by an EKG and an x-ray. Getting blood drawn was a little scary but the edge was taken off by the phlebotomist who had shoes that squeaked against the floor just like Squidward from the cartoon, SpongeBob Square Pants. Having a very good phlebotomist (as we were lucky enough to have this time) makes a significant difference in the amount of pain endured during a blood drawing.

FENESTRATION CLOSURE

The catheterization went well. They had to abort the first attempt at installing the Star Flex. But the second attempt went just fine. One of the doctors took us into the cath lab after the procedure and played back a series of X-rays of the installation that made it appear as though the procedure was filmed. Needless to say, it was very interesting to watch. As an added bonus, I was able to convince the doctor to give us as a souvenir the Star Flex from the first aborted attempt at installing it.

NOVEMBER 3, 2005

Today is Annie's eighth birthday. She was so excited to go to school today with the cupcakes that she made with her best friend yesterday for their second grade class. She continues to do very well in both physical and mental development. Annie can't wait for the snow to come so that we can go skiing. Finally, she is taking skating lessons this year and is really enjoying it. The first unassisted bike ride happened this summer as well as her learning how to roller blade. Her swimming abilities greatly improved this summer. Golfing isn't quite her thing but she does like "to play on weekends".

I reread this diary today to help recall everything that we went through to get to where we are now. Time has faded the memories of some of the details, but the lesson of not taking things or people for granted will never be forgotten.

The unfortunate aspect of human nature is that we tend to slip back into old habits. As memories fade, we find ourselves worrying about things that just aren't important. The good news is that we are surrounded by things and opportunities that help bring those memories, and with them the lessons learned, back to life.

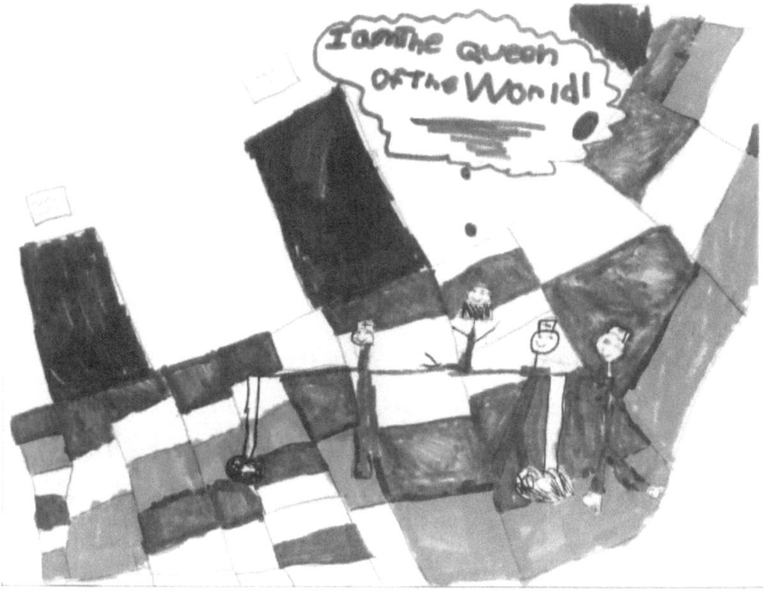

Figure 9: Annie Gets a Free Ride Down the Hall in Her Crib

Strangely enough, Annie, to this day, talks about how much fun it was to be wheeled through the halls of the Hospital in her crib as she was moved from her room to the Cath Lab and back.

A NURSE'S PERSPECTIVE

The following text is a Clinical Exemplar written by one of Annie's primary nurses, Suzanne Murphy McDonough, and submitted to the head of the ICU nursing staff. A Clinical Exemplar is included with each nurse's annual evaluation in which the nurse is asked to write about a patient/family experience and how their efforts impacted this patient/family. It was written shortly after Annie's first birthday. In the Exemplar, Annie is referred to as, "AMS", in order to protect patient identity. The Exemplar is included here to provide a nurse's perspective of some of the events that took place.

AMS was a full term baby girl, prenatally diagnosed with PA/IVS.[1] Her parents were a professional couple, who had had numerous visits with their Cardiologist and Cardiac Surgeon before AMS was born. I started caring for AMS the morning after she had been born and had been admitted to P6 (the Cardiovascular Intensive Care Unit). We needed to take AMS to the cath lab to further explore her cardiac anatomy. I met her parents and her aunt after we had returned from the cath lab, and just before they were to meet with the Cardiac Surgeon. Mom and the aunt were tearful and anxious. Dad was quiet. We spent some time talking about what we were doing for AMS and what to expect in the next hours and days. I tried

1. Pulmonary Atresia/Intact Ventricular Septum

to find positive things to say about their new daughter, while Mom seemed to be able to only focus on her surviving surgery and getting home. She didn't seem able to think beyond the moment for her daughter. She wouldn't allow herself to think of, or hope for her daughter beyond this moment. As much as they had been prepared, they still were not ready for this and terribly fearful of losing their daughter, which Mom easily communicated. Shortly thereafter, the Cardiac Surgeon came in and reviewed AMS's cath results with her parents. He very matter-of-factly explained that her diagnosis was more serious than he had previously explained in their prenatal visits. "Not the news I had expected." "It puts her at the worst end of the spectrum for patients with Pulmonary Atresia", I remember him saying. The news just stunned everyone- myself included. "This will increase the risks of operating on AMS and lower her chances of survival", the Surgeon went on to say. AMS's parents calmly and methodically asked questions regarding their daughter's surgery the next day. After the Surgeon left their bed space, they all wept openly, but separately– Mom quietly by the isolette, the Dad and Aunt pacing around the bed space. I didn't know which family member to console first. I also felt a bit confused as to whether I should try to talk to them at this moment, as they seemed to want some privacy. After some time, AMS's mom motioned me over to the isolette. She asked a few more questions, apologized for crying, and informed me that they were returning to her room on the Maternity Ward at the

Birthing Hospital. I took this opportunity to talk about what they might be feeling. I assured her that there was no need for an apology and that I had hoped they had not viewed my distance as insincerity, but respect for their privacy. She stated she was grateful and thanked me. After the parents left, their Cardiologist called and I informed her of their conversation with the Surgeon and the reaction the parents had had to his news. She too was surprised by the cath report but was more hopeful than the Surgeon. The Cardiologist asked if the parents wanted to speak with her. I ran and caught them at the elevator and AMS's mom came back in to speak, on the phone, with the Cardiologist. They spoke for several minutes. AMS's mom very gratefully thanked me for coming to get her and allowing her to speak with the Cardiologist. She said it helped so much to leave the hospital after speaking with their Cardiologist and hearing her be a little more optimistic-"It's always better to leave on an upbeat note", AMS's mom said as she left.

The parents came in early the next morning and held AMS before she went to surgery. AMS made it through surgery, though she was quite sick postoperatively, requiring much ventilatory and inotropic support. The next day, Dad asked me, "What is the purpose of the whiteboard hanging on the wall?" I told him that sometimes they were used for teaching but for the most part, they went unused. Dad came up with an idea. He would note AMS's "accomplishments of the day" and post them on the whiteboard—the birth of "The Rally Board."

Through our many conversations, the parents were well versed on the "roller-coaster experience" of being a parent with a child in the CICU.[1] They had come to know that there would be "good days and bad days"- and good was sometimes defined as, "nothing bad happened". From that first postop day, until the day AMS was transferred to 6East, where she would continue her recovery, Dad would update the rally board every evening, about 6pm, before the change of (nursing) shift. Some of the ICU staff commented on how odd they found "The Rally Board". I thought it was great in that it gave the Dad something to do, to feel in charge of, and more importantly, to emphasize the positive things going on with AMS. Often he would ask me for help, at which time I'd rib him about his inability to do this on his own. I think this "Rally Board" provided a wonderful outlet for this family and I found myself encouraging other families to do the same. Over the next two weeks AMS made slow, but steady, progress. As we soon came to note, AMS had her own agenda and did things at her own speed. Slowly as AMS overcame the hurdles of an ICU stay, her mom allowed herself to talk of a future with her daughter. Her mom and I found it easy to talk. We had found a common bond beyond that of a nurse caring for her daughter, but of two professional working mothers of two small children. We shared childcare and childrearing stories, and we became friends. She often

---

1. Cardiovascular Intensive Care Unit

thanked me for my support and words of encouragement.

On the day AMS was transferred out of the CICU, Dad took a picture of "The Rally Board", noting the accomplishment of the day: "TRANSFERRED TO 6EAST!!!!!" During AMS's stay at Children's, Dad would also use the Internet daily to update all of their family, friends and colleagues. The feedback they got was a tremendous source of support. One day, AMS's mom was inundated with phone calls and visits from a multitude of friends, only to discover a computer printout left lying on the bedside stand. It seemed that AMS's dad had requested, via the Internet, calls and visits from their family and friends while he had to travel out of town on business. He didn't want his wife to be left alone, without any support. The response was so tremendous that AMS's mom had to take the phone off the hook and lead her many visitors down the hall to a bigger visiting area. She showed me the Internet request for help. It was very sweet. Dad was trying to take care of everything even from miles away. He was always so concerned about his wife. One evening, he came over to P6 to see me and thank me for taking such good care of his wife and helping her through such a difficult time. "She couldn't have done it without you" he said. I thanked him for his kind words. After a few weeks in the hospital, AMS was finally ready to go home. They were nervous, about leaving the security of the hospital, but they were oh so ready to celebrate the holidays with their beautiful daughter at home.

A few weeks passed and it was the morning of Christmas Eve. I was busily running around my house getting last minute holiday things done, when the doorbell rang. There was a "special delivery" for me, the FedEx Man said. I opened up the box to find the most wonderful gift of thanks from AMS and her family. I opened a beautifully wrapped package which I discovered contained a gorgeous Halcyon Days enamel box. It was adorned with roses, lilies and butterflies. Inside the box, an inscription read: "I will bring little children with me who will pretend to be fairies ...and butterflies." Under the box, I discovered a Christmas card with the sweetest picture of my little AMS and her big brother holding her lovingly. Seeing this picture of this sweet little baby, now at home with her family, I was moved to tears. But that was not the end of the surprises. Tucked inside the Christmas card, I discovered some computer printouts. AMS's parents had included four pages of Internet messages to me from some of the people they had been corresponding with since AMS's birth. At first I didn't quite understand what I was reading. But then I discovered that these notes were addressed to me. They were full of thanks and praise for my caring for AMS and her parents. The notes were from family and friends- all people I had never met before, yet they wrote the most sincere and personal things. They relayed their own personal experiences with nurses-one compared me to an angel. The tears were flowing long before I finished the first page of notes. One note was especially touching as it was written by a mother of a baby girl who had died in our unit, about the experienced they had with their nurse-one of my friends. I was overwhelmed by the time I finished the last page. I have always prided myself in taking very good care of my patients and their families, but now I was reading about it, through someone else's eyes. It was amazing! These letters were truly the most tremendous thank-you I have ever received, and I will treasure them always.

CONCLUSION

We still find ourselves anxious to meet and talk with those who have successfully gone down this path before us. Recently, Annie attended a birthday party at a local rock climbing facility. Coincidentally and unbeknownst to us, one of the staff was the much older patient that Annie shared a lecture hour with allowing a group of first-year medical students an opportunity to ask questions of two actual patients. Even though it had been a few years since the lecture hour, he recognized Annie's name on the waiver form and called the contact number to re-establish contact with us. It was great to hear from him and comforting to us to know that he is doing well.

Both his and Annie's successes represent hope. The more contact we can promote amongst those with similar experiences, the better we will all be. We hope that by making our experience public, we can help others who are about to embark on a similar experience by showing them an example of what they can expect – both good and bad. Help us pass hope along by telling others about this book and visiting us at:

www.erallyboard.com.

Focusing on seemingly insignificant progress hidden by overwhelmingly negative circumstances is how we managed to get through this experience. The Rally Board became the vehicle for maintaining that focus. Hopefully, this book will help others maintain focus on small progress by whatever means works best for them.

Made in United States
Troutdale, OR
11/03/2026

56852533R00050